DIABETIC COOKBOOK FOR CHILDREN

A COMPLETE COOKBOOK WITH MEAL PLAN FOR DIABETIC KIDS

BY

JOYCE LIFTED

COPYRIGHT

All rights reserved. No part of this publication may be republished in any form or by any means, including translation, scanning, photocopying, etc., without the prior written permission of the copyright owner.

Table of Contents

INTRODUCTION

The book diabetic cookbook for children aims to give an overview of diabetes and its impact on children, as well as the significance of proper nutrition in managing diabetes in children. It also provides an overview of the cookbook and its purpose. Diabetes is a habitual condition characterized by high situations of sugar (glucose) in the blood. It occurs when the body is unfit to produce enough insulin or is unfit to use insulin effectively. There are two main types of diabetes type 1 and type 2. Type 1 diabetes is an autoimmune complaint in which the body's vulnerable system attacks and destroys the cells that produce insulin. Type 2 diabetes, on the other hand, is the most common type and is generally caused by life factors similar as being fat, lack of physical exertion and unhealthy diet. Children with diabetes need to manage their blood sugar situations through a combination of drug, physical exertion, and proper nutrition. A diet that's high in fiber, low in fat and sugar, and includes a variety of fruits, vegetables, and whole grains is essential for managing diabetes in children. The purpose of this cookbook is to give families with diabetic children with a variety of succulent and healthy fashions that they can make at home. These fashions are designed to be low in sugar and high in fiber, making them ideal for children with diabetes. The cookbook also includes tips for mess planning and operation, as well as strategies for covering blood sugar situations. The end is to help families make healthy and succulent refection's for their diabetic children and to make managing diabetes a little easier. By the end of this cookbook, families will have a variety of fashions to choose from that cater to the requirements of diabetic children and help them maintain a healthy diet. This cookbook will be a precious resource for families with diabetic children, helping them to make healthy, delicious refection's that can be enjoyed by everyone.

CHAPTER 1:

Breakfast Recipes

This chapter of the diabetic cookbook for children focuses on providing a variety of breakfast recipes that are suitable for children with diabetes. The recipes in this chapter are designed to be low in sugar and high in fiber, making them ideal for managing blood sugar levels.

THE BREAKFAST RECIPES ARE AS FOLLOWS;

Diabetic-Friendly Pancake Recipe:
This recipe uses whole wheat flour, which is high in fiber and helps to regulate blood sugar levels. It also uses a sugar substitute, such as Stevia, to sweeten the pancakes instead of

traditional sugar. Additionally, the recipe includes options for adding in healthy ingredients like berries or banana, which provides added nutrients and fiber.

How to Prepare a Diabetic-Friendly Pancake Recipe;

Ingredients:

1 cup all-purpose flour

1 tablespoon sugar substitute

2 teaspoons baking powder

1/4 teaspoon salt

1 cup unsweetened almond milk

1 egg

1 teaspoon vanilla extract

1 tablespoon vegetable oil

Instructions:

In a large mixing bowl, combine the flour, sugar substitute, baking powder, and salt.

In a separate bowl, whisk together the almond milk, egg, vanilla extract, and vegetable oil.

Include the wet source to the dry source and stir until its get mixed.

Stem a non-stick skillet or griddle over low temperature heat.

Use a ladle to pour 1/4 cup of batter onto the skillet for each pancake.

Cook until bubbles form on the surface and the edges start to look set, about 2-3 minutes.

Carefully flip the pancake and cook for an additional 1-2 minutes on the other side.

Repeat with remaining batter. Serve warm and enjoy!

Note: You can use sugar-free syrup or fresh fruits to top the pancakes.

Diabetic-Friendly Breakfast Burrito Recipe: This recipe uses whole wheat tortillas, which are high in fiber, and a variety of vegetables, such as peppers and onions, to add flavor and nutrition. Instead of using high-fat meats, this recipe suggests using lean proteins like turkey or chicken, and it also uses low-fat cheese to keep the fat content in check.

HOWTO PREPARE A DIABETIC-FRIENDLY BREAKFAST BURRITO RECIPE;

Ingredients:

4 low-carb, high-fiber tortillas

4 eggs

1/4 cup diced onion

1/4 cup diced bell pepper

1/4 cup diced tomato

1/4 cup diced mushrooms

Salt and pepper, to taste

1/4 cup shredded cheddar cheese

1/4 cup salsa

Instructions:

Heat a large skillet over medium heat and add a small amount of oil or non-stick cooking spray.

Crack the eggs into the skillet and scramble until cooked through.

Add the diced onion, bell pepper, tomato, and mushrooms to the skillet. Heat it until the vegetables are softened, for about 5-7 minutes.

Season the egg and vegetable mixture with salt and pepper to taste.

Lay out the tortillas on a clean surface. Divide the egg and vegetable mixture among the tortillas, placing it in the center of each one.

Sprinkle shredded cheese over the top of the egg and vegetable mixture.

Roll the tortillas tightly to form burritos, tucking in the sides to keep the filling inside.

Heat a skillet over medium-high heat. Add the burritos to the skillet and cook until golden brown on each side.

Serve warm and garnish with salsa.

Note: You can also add some cooked lean meat like chicken breast or turkey breast to add some more protein in the breakfast burrito.

Diabetic-Friendly Oatmeal Recipe:
that is high in fiber and provides a slow release of energy to help control blood sugar levels. This recipe includes options for adding in fruits and nuts for added flavor and nutrition.

How to prepare diabetic-friendly oatmeal recipes;

Ingredients:

1 cup rolled oats

2 cups unsweetened almond milk or other non-dairy milk

1/4 cup diced apple

1/4 cup diced pear

1/4 cup raisins

1/4 teaspoon ground cinnamon

1 tablespoon chopped walnuts

1 tablespoon chia seeds

1 tablespoon ground flaxseed

1 teaspoon vanilla extract

1 teaspoon honey or sugar substitute

Instructions:

In a medium saucepan, bring the almond milk to a simmer over medium heat.

Add the rolled oats, diced apple, diced pear, raisins, and ground cinnamon to the saucepan.

Reduce the heat to low and let the oatmeal simmer for 5-7 minutes, or until the oats are cooked through and the fruit is softened.

Remove the saucepan from the heat and stir in the chopped walnuts, chia seeds, ground flaxseed, vanilla extract and honey or sugar substitute.

Serve the oatmeal warm and enjoy.

Note: You can also add some more nuts, seeds, or dried fruits to the oatmeal to add some more flavor and nutrients.

Also, you can use a sugar-free sweetener of your choice instead of honey or sugar substitute.

In summary, this chapter provides a variety of breakfast recipes that are suitable for children with diabetes. These recipes are designed to be low in sugar and high in fiber, making them ideal for managing blood sugar levels. These recipes are not only delicious but also nutritious, providing children with the energy and nutrients they need to start the day.

CHAPTER 2:

Snack Recipes

This chapter of the diabetic cookbook for children focuses on providing a variety of snack recipes that are suitable for children with diabetes. The recipes in this chapter are designed to be low in sugar and high in fiber, making them ideal for managing blood sugar levels between meals.

THE SNACK RECIPES PROVIDED IN THIS CHAPTER ARE;

Diabetic-Friendly Smoothie Recipe: This recipe uses a combination of fruits, such as berries, and vegetables, such as spinach, to provide a variety of nutrients and fiber. It also uses a sugar substitute, such as Stevia, to sweeten the smoothie instead of traditional sugar, and it uses a low-fat milk or yogurt as a base. This recipe is easy to make, and it can be a great option for children who are on the go.

HOW TO PREPARE DIABETIC-FRIENDLY SMOOTHIE RECIPE;

Ingredients:

1 cup unsweetened almond milk or other non-dairy milk

1/2 cup frozen berries (such as blueberries, raspberries, or blackberries)

1/2 banana

1/4 avocado

1 tablespoon ground flaxseed

1 teaspoon honey or sugar substitute

1 teaspoon vanilla extract

1 scoop protein powder (optional)

Instructions:

In a blender, combine the almond milk, frozen berries, banana, avocado, ground flaxseed, honey or sugar substitute, vanilla extract, and protein powder (if using).

Blend the ingredients on high speed until smooth and creamy.

Taste the smoothie and adjust the sweetness as needed.

Pour the smoothie into a glass and enjoy.

Note: You can also add some spinach or kale for added nutrition, or switch up the fruit to use whatever you have on hand.

You can use sugar-free sweetener of your choice instead of honey or sugar substitute.

Also, you can use Greek yogurt instead of avocado to make it creamier, it will add some more protein to the smoothie.

Diabetic-Friendly Yogurt Parfait Recipe: This recipe uses low-fat Greek yogurt as a base, which is high in protein and low in sugar. It also includes options for adding in fruits, nuts, and seeds for added flavor and nutrition. This recipe is a great option for children who are looking for a healthy and satisfying snack.

HOW TO PREPARE A DIABETIC-FRIENDLY YOGURT PARFAIT RECIPE;

Ingredients:

1 cup plain Greek yogurt

1/4 cup fresh berries (such as blueberries, raspberries, or blackberries)

2 tablespoons unsweetened shredded coconut

2 tablespoons chopped nuts (such as almonds, walnuts, or pecans)

2 tablespoons honey or sugar substitute

1 teaspoon vanilla extract

Instructions:

In a bowl, mix together the Greek yogurt, honey or sugar substitute, and vanilla extract until well combined.

In a separate bowl, toss the fresh berries with 1 tablespoon of honey or sugar substitute.

To assemble the parfait, layer the yogurt mixture, berries, shredded coconut, and chopped nuts in a jar or glass. Repeat the layers until the jar are filled, ending with a layer of yogurt mixture.

Garnish with additional berries and shredded coconut, if desired.

Serve chilled and enjoy.

Note: You can use any kind of fresh or frozen fruits you like or have on hand; you can also add some granola or muesli for added texture and flavor.

You can use sugar-free sweetener of your choice instead of honey or sugar substitute.

Also, you can add some chia seeds or flaxseed to add some more fiber and healthy fats to the parfait.

Diabetic-Friendly Trail Mix Recipe that is high in fiber and protein, which helps to control blood sugar levels. This recipe includes a variety of nuts and seeds, such as almonds and pumpkin seeds, as well as dried fruits like cranberries or apricots. It also uses a sugar substitute, such as Stevia, to sweeten the trail mix, instead of traditional sugar.

HOW TO PREPAR DIABETIC-FRIENDLY TRAIL MIX RECIPE;

Ingredients:

1 cup unsalted roasted almonds

1/2 cup unsalted roasted sunflower seeds

1/2 cup unsweetened dried cranberries or other dried fruit

1/4 cup unsweetened shredded coconut

1/4 cup dark chocolate chips or cacao nibs

1 tablespoon honey or sugar substitute

1 teaspoon ground cinnamon

Instructions:

In a large mixing bowl, combine the almonds, sunflower seeds, dried cranberries or other dried fruit, shredded coconut, chocolate chips or cacao nibs, honey or sugar substitute, and ground cinnamon.

Mix well to combine all the ingredients.

Take the mixture out on baking zinc lined with parchment paper.

Bake in a preheated 350F/175C oven for 10-15 minutes or until the nuts and seeds are toasted and fragrant.

Take it away from the oven and allow it to get cool.

Once cooled, store the trail mix in an airtight container for up to 2 weeks.

Enjoy as a snack, a topping for yogurt or oatmeal, or add it to your favorite trail mix recipe.

Note: You can use any kind of nuts and seeds you like, you can also add some pumpkin seeds, or flax seeds, or sesame seeds.

You can use sugar-free sweetener of your choice instead of honey or sugar substitute.

Also, you can add some spices like nutmeg or ginger to add some more flavors to the trail mix.

In summary, this chapter provides a variety of snack recipes that are suitable for children with diabetes. These recipes are designed to be low in sugar and high in fiber, making them ideal for managing blood sugar levels between meals. These recipes are not only delicious but also nutritious, providing children with the energy and nutrients they need to get through the day. They are also easy to make, portable and can be a great option for children who are on the go.

CHAPTER 3:

Lunch and Dinner Recipes

We will focus on providing a variety of lunch and dinner recipes that are suitable for children with diabetes. The recipes in this chapter are designed to be low in sugar and high in fiber, making them ideal for managing blood sugar levels throughout the day.

One of the lunch and dinner recipes provided in this chapter is a diabetic-friendly grilled chicken recipe. This recipe uses lean protein such as skinless chicken breast, which is low in fat and high in protein, it also marinates the chicken in a combination of herbs and spices, which add flavor without adding sugar. Additionally, the recipe suggests serving the chicken with a side of vegetables, such as broccoli or green beans, which provide added fiber and nutrition.

Another lunch and dinner recipe in this chapter is a diabetic-friendly fish taco recipe. This recipe uses a variety of vegetables, such as peppers, onions, and cabbage, to add flavor and nutrition. The fish used in the recipe is a low-fat fish, like tilapia or cod, and it is also seasoned with a variety of herbs and spices. Instead of using traditional high-carb tortillas, this recipe suggests using lettuce leaves or low-carb tortillas as a wrap for the tacos.

Lastly, the chapter includes a diabetic-friendly quinoa and black bean salad recipe that is high in fiber and protein, which helps to control blood sugar levels. This recipe includes a variety of vegetables, such as bell peppers, tomatoes, and corn, as well as a combination of quinoa and black beans, which provide a great balance of carbohydrates and protein. It also uses a combination of herbs and spices, such as cumin and chili powder, to add flavor without adding sugar.

In summary, we provide a variety of lunch and dinner recipes that are suitable for children with diabetes.

These recipes are designed to be low in sugar and high in fiber, making them ideal for managing blood sugar levels throughout the day. These recipes are not only delicious but also nutritious, providing children with the energy and nutrients they need to get through the day. They also include a balance of carbohydrates, protein, and healthy fats, which can be important for a diabetic diet.

CHAPTER 4:

Dessert Recipes

Dessert recipes are suitable for children with diabetes. The recipes in this chapter are designed to be low in sugar and high in fiber, making them ideal for managing blood sugar levels while still allowing children to enjoy a sweet treat.

One of the dessert recipes provided in this chapter is a diabetic-friendly berry sorbet recipe. This recipe uses a combination of frozen berries, such as strawberries and blueberries, and a sugar substitute, such as Stevia, to sweeten the sorbet instead of traditional sugar. Berries are naturally low in sugar and high in fiber, making them a great option for a diabetic-friendly dessert.

Another dessert recipe in this chapter is a diabetic-friendly chocolate chip cookie recipe. This recipe uses whole wheat flour, which is high in fiber and helps to regulate blood sugar levels. It also uses a sugar substitute, such as Stevia, to sweeten the cookies instead of traditional sugar, and it uses a combination of healthy fats, such as coconut oil or almond butter, instead of traditional butter.

Lastly, the chapter includes a diabetic-friendly apple crisp recipe that is high in fiber and low in sugar. This recipe uses a combination of apples, such as granny smith and honey crisp, and a sugar substitute, such as Stevia, to sweeten the apple crisp instead of traditional sugar. It also uses a combination of whole wheat flour and oats, which provide a great balance of carbohydrates and protein, to make the crisp topping.

In summary, this chapter provides a variety of dessert recipes that are suitable for children with diabetes. These recipes are designed to be low in sugar and high in fiber, making them ideal for managing blood sugar levels while still allowing children to enjoy a sweet treat. These recipes are not only delicious but also nutritious, providing children with the energy and nutrients they need to get through the day. They are also easy to make, and they can be a great option for children who are looking for a sweet treat that is not too high in sugar.

CHAPTER 5:

Meal Planning and Management

The tips and strategies for planning and preparing diabetic-friendly refection's isn't to outlook beget It'll also provides guidelines for covering blood sugar situations in the life of any diabetic kiddies. Thus, the tips are as follows; it suggests preparing refection's in advance, similar as on the weekends, so that they can be fluently reheated during the week. This can save time and make it easier for families to stick to a diabetic-friendly diet.   Another tip is for managing portion sizes. It suggests using lower plates and measuring out serving sizes to help control the quantum of food consumed. This can be especially important for children with diabetes, as portion control is an important aspect of managing blood sugar situations.

Guideline for Monitoring Sugar Level It suggests checking blood sugar situations ahead and after refections, as well as ahead and after physical exertion. It also suggests keeping a log of blood sugar situations, which can be participated with a healthcare provider to help track progress and make any necessary adaptations to the treatment plan.

Here's a sample meal roster for a diabetic child:

Breakfast:

Scrambled eggs with diced vegetables and whole wheat toast

Greek yogurt with fresh berries and a drizzle of honey or sugar substitute

Oatmeal with diced fruit and chopped nuts

Snack:

Baby carrots and hummus

Apple slices with almond butter

Trail mix made with unsalted nuts and seeds, dried fruit, and dark chocolate chips or cacao nibs

Lunch:

Turkey and cheese sandwich on whole wheat bread with lettuce and tomato

Grilled chicken breast with steamed vegetables and quinoa

Whole wheat pasta together with turkey meatballs and marinara sauce.

Snack:

String cheese

Rice cakes with peanut butter

Diabetic-friendly smoothie made with non-dairy milk, frozen berries, and ground flaxseed

Dinner:

Bake fish together with a side of roasted green leaves.

Diabetic-friendly pancakes with turkey bacon and fresh fruit.

Whole wheat pizza with vegetables and lean protein (such as chicken or turkey)

Snack:

Yogurt parfait made with plain Greek yogurt, fresh berries, and unsweetened shredded coconut

Air-popped popcorn with a sprinkle of nutritional yeast and sea salt

Diabetic-friendly trail mix made with unsalted nuts, seeds, and dried fruit.

Note: It's important to consult with a healthcare professional, such as a pediatric endocrinologist, dietitian or a doctor to create an individualized meal plan that works best for the child. The child's activity level, medication regimen, and blood glucose targets must be considered.

In summary, this chapter provides tips and strategies for planning and preparing diabetic-friendly refections, as well as guidelines for covering blood sugar situations. It's an important chapter for families with diabetic children, as it helps them to understand the significance of planning and medication in managing diabetes.

The tips and guidelines handed in this chapter will empower families to take control of their child's diabetes and make healthy choices that will help keep blood sugar situations in check.

Here is the sample meal roster for a diabetic child;

Breakfast; authority, and blood glucose targets must be considered.

Conclusion

It is important for families to understand that managing diabetes is a lifelong commitment, but with the help of this cookbook, they now have the resources to make delicious and healthy meals for their children. The recipes and tips provided in this cookbook can be easily adapted to fit the unique needs and preferences of each child and family.

In conclusion, this cookbook is a valuable resource for families with diabetic children, helping them to make healthy, tasty meals that can be enjoyed by everyone. It is a reminder that a diabetes diagnosis does not have to mean the end of enjoying delicious food, and that with proper planning, preparation and monitoring, managing diabetes can be manageable.